REBRAND YOUR LIFE: DRINKS THAT WILL BOOST METABOLISM FOR WEIGHT LOSS IN 28 DAYS

by

JANET SMITH

Dedicated to all my readers

Other books by Janet Smith

The Complete Ketogenic Diet For Starters: Essential Guide To Keto Lifestyle: Low Carbs, More Energy

Tested And Trusted: Newly Found Recipes That Will Help You Lose Weight In 4 Weeks: Burn Fat While Eating

Poached Eggs: These Little Secrets Mean A Lot

Total Eating Guide: Easiest Way To Trim Down In 28 Days, Stay Healthy And Live Longer

28 Days Weight Loss Plan: Don't Starve. Don't Suffer Counting Calories: Eat These New Fast Metabolism Diets: Your Journey To Trimming Down

Table of Contents

- SLIMMING KALE AND ACV DRINK
- WHEATGRASS AND GRAPE FAT MOBILIZER
- TONING WHEY PROTEIN AND CHIA SEED DRINK
- WEIGHT LOSS LEMONADE
- SKINNY CINNAMON AND PAPAYA DRINK

INTRODUCTION

Have you ever thought there are drinks that will help you lose weight? If yes, kudos to you. You're one step up the ladder. It is a fact that what goes inside reflects on the outside. This book, seeks to assist people improve their health, by virtue of what they drink. The drinks discussed can go a long way in improving your health and managing overweight. More so, the recipes are easy to follow. Why not begin now, to drink something that will help you live long?

As you follow the instructions in this book, you will trim off excess pounds of flesh, and be better able to cope with stress and any element that might hamper your quality life. Good health to you.

CHAPTER ONE

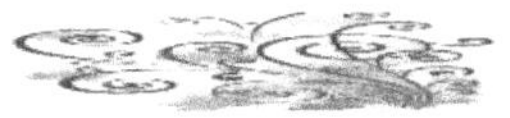

PEAR JUICE

I work really hard trying to ensure our restaurant business is up and doing. I attend to clients on my ketogenic diet plan. I help people who're interested in workouts for weight loss. I also write books. Like this one you are reading. The very good thing about this particular book is that my clients believe it is easier to follow than the meal plans. One woman wrote me a mail after reading an article on weight loss on my site. She said: 'As regards your article on drinks for metabolism, this is easy and effective.'

She was sincere and I thought I should perhaps write a book on this. Now that you're reading this book, I'm hopeful you'll see great results after following the recipes. Two of the drinks and their recipes discussed in the final chapter of this book actually helped that lady who sent me a mail.

However, I chose to start with pear juice because I had formerly undermined its effect until early in 2018 when a fellow nutritionist told me her client trimmed down with pear juice in the plan. Why am I saying all these? I want you to take the information in this book seriously. I can guarantee you of great results.

Really, there are a lot of drinks out there that will help you lose weight. In this book, you'd appreciate the scientific proofs why the drinks are effective. But why did I include pear juice in this? Well, you'll see for yourself.

Simply speaking, any drink made with pear as the major ingredient is pear juice. Some may decide to add milk and a bit of honey to improve on the look. While there those who really like it when mango and pineapple is crushed with it in the electric juicer. However, before I go on to tell you the 'how to', take some time to look at the health benefits packed inside pear juice,

Benefits of taking pear juice

Pear juice is not a commonly known drink. But it is quite tasty. If you give it a try, you will always want it again. Some of the benefits of drinking pear juice include;

1. Low caloric content:

The common complaint that people have about other fruit juice is the high caloric content in them which is obtained from natural sugars. But pears are among the foods with the lowest calorie. An average pear juice contains about 58 calories (just one glass). The nutrition provided by pears is quite immeasurable and it gives you a feeling of satisfaction. So people who desire to lose weight can add pears to their diet. It is both a high-energy and high- nutrient food with little impact on weight gain.

2. Maintaining the skin:

If you want to prevent premature aging, pear juice is right for you. Pear fruit has high a high amount of Vitamin C, copper and Vitamin K. These nutrients give the fruit juice the ability to fight harmful radicals and thus protect the skin cells from damage. There is toning of the skin and the formation of lines near the eyes and lip area is prevented or stopped.

3. Prevention of cancer:

One health benefit of pear juice is that it can prevent the development of cancer. The fibers from pear juice can bind themselves with bile acids and a special group of bile acids known as secondary bile acids. The high amounts of secondary bile acids present in our intestines can increase the risk of colorectal cancer. But the fiber in pear helps to reduce the concentration in the intestine, and lower the risk of developing cancer. Taking pear juice also reduces the risk of stomach cancer. The various key components in fiber phytonutrients and cinnamic acids have cancer fighting properties. A study done in Mexico City showed that 2 fruit servings of pear can decrease the risk of gastric cancer. Esophageal cancer is a dangerous type of cancer but pear juice can reduce the risk and effect. A large scale study was done by the National Institute of Health and American

Association of Retired persons, which showed that pear was a key food that reduced the risk of esophageal cancer.

4. Antioxidant activity:

Pears contain a good amount of antioxidants just like other fruits. These antioxidants are helpful in fighting various diseases and illnesses in the body. Antioxidants help eliminate the free radicals which gather in the body through a process called cellular metabolism. These free radicals can change healthy DNA into cancerous cells which can have a devastating effect. So the antioxidant components of Vitamin A, Vitamin C, and beta-carotene which are found in pear juice can help the body get rid of dangerous diseases.

5. Digestive and intestinal health:

Pear juice has an important role in digestion. One glass of pear juice provides about 18% of the daily body requirement of fiber which are a strong agent for digestive health and function. The majority fiber in pear is non-soluble polysaccharide. This means it acts as a bulking agent in the intestines. It gathers the food and adds bulk to it so that the food can easily pass through the intestines. It also stimulates the secretion of gastric and digestive juices so that the food can move smoother in a digested state. More so, bowel movement is put under control thus reducing the chances of constipation.

The pear juice also binds itself to the cancer- causing and free radicals in the colon and helps to protect the organ from harmful effects. It is noteworthy that Pear juice has about 6.5% fructose and 1.3% sucrose. Free fructose isn't absorbed properly. It becomes fermented in the large intestines thus resulting in the production of SCFA (Short chained fatty acid) which leads to the absorption of a small energy in the colon. This explains why we use pear juices in the treatment of constipation.

6. Birth defects:

Folate is another valuable nutritional components found in pear juice. Research has shown that folic acid correlates positively with the reduction of neural tube defects in newborns. So, pregnant women are encouraged to drink pear juice.

7. Potassium content:

Pear juice is a good source of potassium. Potassium is a good vasodilator (it opens the blood vessels). It helps to lower the blood pressure and the strain on cardiovascular system and thus stops the formation of clots. It also increases the blood flow to all parts of the body. Low blood pressure leads to lower chances of different cardiovascular diseases like strokes, atherosclerosis, and heart attacks. Potassium also helps to regulate the fluids in the body and keeps different organs hydrated.

8. Bone health:

Pear juices contain minerals in high amount. These minerals include phosphorous, manganese, magnesium, copper and calcium. This means that the effects of bone loss and serious bone conditions like osteoporosis and general weakness of the body are reduced.

9. Skin, eyes and hair:

Vitamin A is one of the most important vitamins in the body. Pears have high amount of vitamin A and other components like leutin and zea-xanthin. They function as a good antioxidant and reduce the effects of aging on skin. Pear juice also reduces hair loss, cataracts and other health conditions that come with aging.

10.　　　For weaning children:

Pear juice is so helpful for weaning children (stopping the supply of breast milk and introducing a young child to an adult's diet). The reason is that it is hypoallergenic. So it doesn't result in any digestion problems. The fruit juice can be served cold to children. But it shouldn't be given to children with diarrhea.

How to make Pear juice:

Pear juice can be made with an electric juicer. The juicer makes it easy for you to experiment with different flavors for pears. Here is how to make some delicious pear juice at home:

1. You should select firm and bright pears, with skin that is free of bruises and imperfections. Firm pears produce better juice. You will end up making a puree when the pears are too soft.

2. Ensure to wash the pears in cold water. Wash the surface area to remove any kind of dirt.

3. At this point you will need to cut the pear and remove any seeds and stem attached to it. Cut the pear into little chunks before you put into the electric juicer. (Chop any other ingredients you want to put with pear juice.). You can add fruits like pineapple, mango, apple and vegetables like celery, spinach, broccoli and carrots.

4. Put additional ingredients into the juicer and run the juicer. I usually enjoy adding a lot of condensed milk to enhance the taste.

At this point, you can remove the juice compartment and serve the pear juice. Enjoy the pear juice fresh.

How Best To Store:

The best way to store pear juice is to put it in a refrigerator. You may wish to use an air tight container, freezer bag, Mason jar, or ice cube tray.

When the pear juice is taken out of storage, it might be a bit thicker. You may dilute it with a lighter drink or water. You can also defrost the juice and make pear jellies.

CHAPTER TWO

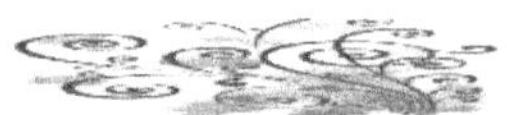

COFFEE

Let me ask you; do you really know coffee? I'm sure you are probably nodding or smiling by now. But then what do you know about coffee? Do you know that around the world, countless numbers of people prefer to start the day with a warm cup of coffee? I take coffee in the morning too. But when I was studying for a bachelor's, I would drink a cup of coffee at night to keep me alert during night studies. Drinking coffee is a great way to get together with family and friends! Can you imagine the joy of sipping up during such friendly atmosphere? It lifts our moods and relieves stress. More so, coffee has an enticing aroma and distinctive flavor (you know what I mean).

But did you know that besides the enticing aroma, reviving taste and distinctive flavor, a cup of coffee contains a solid bunch of health benefits? Let me start by telling you ten reasons why coffee is splendid and absolutely good for you.

Reasons You Should Start Taking Coffee

First of all, Coffee does not interfere with calcium absorption. There is a common misconception that taking coffee can lead to calcium loss from the body. But current study has shown that coffee has no negative effect on bone health. And of course, strong and healthy bones are a result of diets rich in calcium. Why not prepare your coffee with a full glass of milk? This will certainly help you meet your calcium needs.

Second of all, soluble Coffee is 100% coffee. Soluble coffee is processed using pure coffee beans and water without additives. It's the selection of beans and the distinctive roasting process that provides its special aroma.

Third of all, Coffee helps you learn better and stay more alert at work. Studies have proved that people who take coffee are relaxed and more interested in their work. The caffeine content in coffee helps to restore and maintain alertness, thereby improving performance and enhancing your mood. It is the perfect brew if you want to be alert and active at work. When studying, coffee helps improve attention and wakefulness, increasing attentiveness and by that it facilitates learning. (While I was studying for a bachelor's degree, I made a second class upper because Nescafe kept me alert at night; the time I studied best).

Fourth of all, Coffee is the number one source of antioxidants. Current research has shown that coffee contributes significantly to your daily total antioxidant intake. Antioxidants help protect your cells from oxidation and your body from cancer, heart disease, and premature aging!

Fifth of all, Coffee enhances your physical performance. According to research, caffeine plays a role in contributing to better physical performance. This could help athletes perform better at endurance exercises of short and long durations, as well as strenuous routines

Sixth of all, Coffee can help protect your skin. Your skin is constantly exposed to harmful external factors such as UV ray, which can affect the health of your cells and cause them to damage. But with the antioxidant-rich properties of coffee, your skin can fight the damaging effects of the sun and prevent wrinkles as well.

Last of all, Coffee can help ease headaches. Research suggests that a cup of coffee may help to relieve you of migraine symptoms and even stop it if consumed at the very initial stage of the headache. This is because substances like caffeine constrict blood vessels and help counter the throbbing effects of blood vessel dilation in your head.

Whether you choose a caffeinated or decaffeinated blend, you will still get all the benefits of antioxidants since both have similar content. You can drink 3-4 cups a day. For those who take coffee, the recommendation for moderate consumption is 300 mg of caffeine daily or the equivalent of 3-4 cups of soluble coffee. 1 cup of soluble coffee has less than 2 calories. In fact it is what you add to the coffee that adds calories. So remember to have your cup with less sugar and low fat milk.

CHAPTER THREE

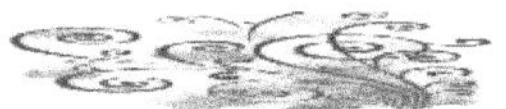

GREEN COFFEE

Green coffee is currently among the world's most popular weight loss supplements. As the name implies, this supplement is extracted from the same beans people use for brewing coffee. The only difference is that green coffee beans are raw, unroasted coffee beans. The roasting process seems to destroy some of the healthy, natural chemicals in the beans. Because of media attention, green coffee has become a popular supplement for weight loss.

Benefit of taking Green coffee:

1. Green coffee also seems to help lower high blood pressure in some people. One small study in people with mild high blood pressure showed benefit over the placebo

2. Some research shows green coffee may help with weight loss. A few small studies found that people taking green coffee lost 3 to 5 pounds more than people who weren't. Green coffee may act by lowering blood sugar and blocking fat buildup.

Quantity of Green coffee to take:

The active ingredients in supplements vary widely from maker to maker. This makes it hard to set a standard dose. Ask your doctor for advice. Before you venture into green coffee, please tell your doctor about any supplements you're taking, even if they're natural. That will help your doctor check on any potential side effects or interactions with medications.

Wait a minute. Have you heard about Coffee beans? Like any other beans they are complex in nature. There are some 40 different substances responsible for the taste and health properties of coffee. However, the main thing I want to tell you relates to Green coffee beans. It is no longer uncommon to hear about Green coffee beans and the health benefit. Green coffee beans are the coffee beans in their natural form. The truth is that these beans are the same coffee beans that you consume daily in the form of drink. The only difference is that Green coffee beans are unroasted. When these beans are later roasted for commercial use, they turn brown and lose Chlorogenic Acid which is largely responsible for weight loss. So if you are looking forward to the weight loss benefit of coffee you should use the green coffee beans in the unroasted form.

The taste of green coffee beans is very much different from the roasted beans that you usually make. The flavor you will get from the green beans is not very strong and hence you will get little watery taste. Those having problems with the taste of green coffee can take green coffee extract because of its improved taste.

It is possible to find the roasted coffee beans around you but to get the fresh green coffee beans; you may need to go online where you will find the best.

Before you make green coffee drink from unroasted coffee beans, keep the following in mind:

- Ensure to use the best quality Arabica coffee beans to get the best taste. You can also use the one grown by organic farming.

- If you are allergic to coffee or have any tolerance issues, please check with your doctor before consuming this drink.

Ingredients for Making Green Coffee:

- Green Coffee Beans (Arabica or similar) 20 g
- Hot water 300 ml or 2 cups
- Honey or sugar (this is optional)

There are two methods for making green coffee drink. Whatever method you want to opt for, just endure that the coffee beans are unroasted.

Method 1–

How to prepare coffee using green coffee bean powder:

- Grind the green coffee beans in a grinder to get the fine powder depending on your liking and the available appliance. Green coffee beans are unroasted beans, so they are really hard to grind. You will require heavy duty grinder.

- Divide the powder into two cups and add in hot water. Water should be hot but not boiling (about 90°C).

- Leave for 10 minutes and then drain with fine sieve to get your drink ready to sip.

- You may add sugar or honey if you like but for those looking for the health benefits; it is recommended to drink it plain.

Method 2-

How to prepare green coffee using whole green coffee beans:

Preparing coffee from whole beans is usually a time consuming method. You may prepare this coffee in large batches. Soak the beans overnight in water.

- Heat the mixture of soaked beans and water. When it is boiled, simmer the mixture on low flame for 15 minutes. Stir occasionally.

- Ensure the mixture is cool before sieving it to remove beans from the mixture.

- The concoction you are now having is concentrated. So you may add filtered or distilled water to dilute the concoction.

- If you have prepared this in a large batch then you can store the rest in a deep freezer to be used within 3 days.

- Add cardamom or any other additives. This will add more taste to this healthy drink.

Whether you use the first or second method, make sure you take one cup after each meal for best results.

As you take Green Coffee for weight loss, you should keep the following facts in mind.

The caffeine in green coffee, just like the caffeine in brewed coffee, can cause stomach upset, headache and anxiety. However, the major health risks associated with drinking green coffee includes:

1. Glaucoma

2. Diabetes

3. High blood pressure

4. Irritable bowel syndrome

4. Osteoporosis

5. Bleeding disorders

Talk to your doctor if you have any medical conditions before using a green coffee supplement. There is no reliable evidence about its safety of green coffee, so it is not recommended for children or for pregnant or nursing mothers.

Green coffee interacts with many medicines. Some of these include stimulants, blood thinners, and medicines for:

1. Menopause

2. Depression

3. Schizophrenia

4. Heart problems

5. Weak bones

6. Lung diseases

ADVICE: Do not take green coffee along with herbal stimulants or other supplements with caffeine.

CHAPTER FOUR

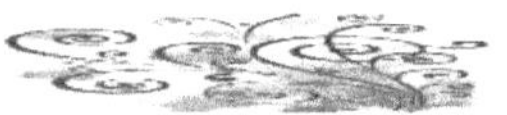

FOURTEEN NEWLY PROVEN DRINKS FOR WEIGHT LOSS

BELLY SHRINK CITRUSY DRINK

What You Will Need

½ cup pomegranate

1 teaspoon organic honey

Pinch of salt

½ cup grapefruit

How to Prepare

1. Add the grapefruit and pomegranates in the blender.

2. Spin and pour it into a glass.

3. Add honey and a pinch of black salt.

4. Stir very well before you begin to enjoy the drink.

What do you stand to benefit from taking this drink?

Grapefruit is quite effective for weight loss. It achieves this by improving insulin sensitivity and post-glucose insulin levels.

Pomegranates work to decrease inflammation and lowers bad cholesterol which directly or indirectly lead to weight loss.

Honey also work to improve your overall body health.

METABOLISM BOOSTING PINEAPPLE DRINK

What You Will Need

½ teaspoon Ceylon cinnamon powder

Pinch of black salt

2½ tablespoon lime juice

1 cup pineapple

How to Prepare

1. Add the pineapple in a blender and blend smoothly.

2. Into a drinking glass, pour the blended pineapple.

3. Add the lime juice, cinnamon powder, and black salt.

4. Stir until you're sure it's well stirred.

What do you stand to benefit from this drink?

Limes are rich in vitamin C, have antioxidant activity, boost immunity, and regulate body weight.

GINGER AND LEMON GUT CLEANSER

What You Will Need

Cup cold water

1 inch ginger root

½ teaspoon roasted cumin powder

½ lime

How to Prepare

1. Chop the ginger and add in a blender.

2. Add the cold water and spin the blender.

3. Pour out the blended mix into a glass.

4. Add roasted cumin powder and lime juice.

5. Stir very well and enjoy the drink.

What do you stand to benefit from this drink?

Limes are rich in vitamin C, have antioxidant activity, boost immunity, and regulate body weight.

SLIMMING GREEN TEA AND MINT

What You Will Need

Cup water

4 or 5 mint leaves

1 tablespoon green tea leaves

How to Prepare

1. Put the mint leaves in a cup of water and bring it to boil.

2. Allow to boil for 5 minutes.

3. Add green tea leaves and allows soaking for an extra 5 minutes.

4. Drain the boiled water into a cup.

5. Stir before drinking.

What do you stand to benefit from this drink?

Green tea contains a catechin called epigallocatechin (EGCG) that aids weight loss by mobilizing fat.

THE FENUGREEK DRINK

What You Will Need

Pinch of salt

2 teaspoon fenugreek seeds

½ cup water

½ cup cucumber

How to Prepare

1. Soak the fenugreek seeds overnight in a half cup of water.

2. Add in the cucumber into a blender and spin.

3. Drain the fenugreek seeds out and pour the water in the blender.

4. Spin and pour into a glass.

5. Add a pinch of black salt and stir very well.

What do you stand to benefit from this drink?

Fenugreek improves glucose and lipid metabolism, increases insulin sensitivity, and has antioxidant properties.

FAST WEIGHT LOSS COCNUT WATER DRINK

What You Will Need

¼ cup pineapple

1 cup coconut water

Pinch of black salt

½ teaspoon ground fennel seeds

How to Prepare

1. Juice the pineapple using a blender.

2. Add the coconut water and ground fennel seeds and spin.

3. Drain the coconut drink into a glass.

4. Add ice before drinking.

What do you stand to benefit from this drink?

Fennel seeds stimulate digestion, prevents bloating, indigestion, and nausea. A clean colon helps in proper absorption of nutrients and helps to flush out toxins resulting in weight loss.

NEGATIVE CALORIE CELERY DRINK

What You Will Need

¼ teaspoons freshly ground black pepper

½ teaspoon apple cider vinegar

½ cup celery

1 cup water

How to Prepare

1. Add the celery in a blender.

2. Pour a cup of water into the blender and spin.

3. Pour the celery juice into a cup and add apple cider vinegar.

4. Stir in the freshly ground black pepper before enjoying the drink.

What do you stand to benefit from taking this drink?

Celery is a negative calorie food. It helps in weight loss by improving lipid metabolism and lowering bad cholesterol levels.

Apple cider vinegar helps weight reduction.

Piperine is an active component of black pepper which helps in weight loss by preventing fat cell proliferation.

TOMATO AND LIME FAT BURNER

What You Will Need

½ lime juice

A cup tomato

Pinch of black salt

How to Prepare

1. Blend the tomatoes in the blender.

2. Pour out the juice in a glass.

3. Add lime juice and a pinch of salt.

4. Stir very well before drinking.

What do you stand to benefit from taking this drink?

Tomatoes are loaded with minerals, vitamins, and phytonutrients that act against obesity, diabetes, hypertension, and cardiovascular disease. Limes are rich in vitamin C, they have antioxidant activity, boost immunity, and regulate body weight.

MORNING HONEY AND LEMON DETOX

What You Will Need

1 ½ tablespoon organic honey

1 ½ lime juice

1 ½ cup water

How to Prepare

1. Heat the water to warm.

2. Add in the lime juice and honey.

3. Stir very well before drinking.

What do I stand to benefit from this drink?

Lemon detox along with a dash of **honey** forms one of the best drinks for weight loss. This is because organic honey helps to prevent gut problems, improve cardiovascular health, and reduces inflammation. This, in turn leads to weight reduction.

Limes are loaded with vitamin C, which helps to boost the immune system, and metabolism for weight loss.

SLIMMING KALE AND ACV DRINK

What You Will Need

1 teaspoon apple cider vinegar (ACV)

½ cup water

1 cup kale

Pinch of black salt

How to Prepare

1. Set the kale into the blender.

2. Add water to the blender and spin.

3. Pour the kale juice into a glass.

4. Mix in apple cider vinegar and a pinch of black salt and stir well before drinking.

What do you stand to benefit from this drink?

Kale is a rich source of antioxidants, dietary fiber, vitamins, and minerals. It helps to reduce the blood glucose levels and therefore can prevent overweight and diabetes.

Apple cider vinegar helps in weight loss and regulates blood pressure.

WHEATGRASS AND GRAPE FAT
MOBILIZER

What You Will Need

2 cups wheatgrass

1 cup grapes

1 cup water

Pinch of black salt

How to Prepare

1. Chop the wheat grass and then toss
    in a Nutribullet.

2. Add in the grapes and water and spin.

3. Pour the juice into a glass.

4. Drain the juice with a sieve (if you use a regular blender).

5. Add a pinch of black salt and mix well.

What do you stand to benefit from this drink?

Wheatgrass helps to lower bad cholesterol, and flush out toxins.

Grapes help to regulate the blood sugar levels, which indirectly aid weight loss.

TONING WHEY PROTEIN AND CHIA SEED DRINK

What You Will Need

2½ tablespoon whey protein

1½ teaspoon chia seeds

1½ cup warm fat-free/soy milk

How to Prepare

1. Add milk, whey protein, and chia seeds into a blender or Nutribullet.

2. Spin the blender.

3. Pour into a glass and enjoy the drink.

What do you stand to benefit from this drink?

Whey protein helps to boosts immunity, and improves cardiovascular health likely resulting in higher metabolism for weight loss

Chia seeds help in weight loss by improving lipid metabolism.

WEIGHT LOSS LEMONADE

What You Will Need

1½ lemon

1½ teaspoon maple syrup

½ teaspoon cayenne pepper

Pinch of salt

How to Prepare

1. Squeeze juice out of lemon into a glass.

2. Add maple syrup and cayenne pepper.

3. Stir very well before drinking.

What do you stand to benefit from this drink?

Lemons are rich in vitamin C and therefore strengthen the immune system against rheumatoid arthritis. Lemons help also in weight loss

Cayenne pepper helps to reduce weight by modulating body metabolism.

SKINNY CINNAMON AND PAPAYA DRINK

What You Will Need

2 cups papaya

1 teaspoon Ceylon cinnamon

2 cups cold water

Pinch of black salt

How to Prepare

1. Blend the papaya with a blender.

2. Mix the cinnamon powder and cold water into a blender and blend again.

3. Empty the papaya drink into a glass.

4. Add a pinch of black salt and stir well.

What do you stand to benefit from this drink?

By improving gut health and lowering cholesterol levels in the blood, **Papaya** helps in weight loss.

Cinnamon has anti-clotting and anti-microbial properties, helps to regulate the blood sugar levels, and improves brain function.\

ABOUT THE AUTHOR

Janet Smith lives with her mother in a small town. They run a restaurant for a living. When she is not at the restaurant, she writes extensively on topics pertaining to food and nutrition.